ESSENTIAL OIL FOR BEGINNERS

By Emily Taylor

The information herein is offered for informational purposes solely, and is universal as so. The presentation of the information is without contract or any type of guarantee assurance.

The trademarks that are used are without any consent, and the publication of the trademark is without permission or backing by the trademark owner. All trademarks and brands within this book are for clarifying purposes only and are the owned by the owners themselves, not affiliated with this document.

Disclaimer and Terms of Use: The Author and Publisher has strived to be as accurate and complete as possible in the creation of this book, notwithstanding the fact that he does not warrant or represent at any time that the contents within are accurate due to the rapidly changing nature of the Internet. While all attempts have been made to verify information provided in this publication, the Author and Publisher assumes no responsibility for errors, omissions, or contrary interpretation of the subject matter herein.

Any perceived slights of specific persons, peoples, or organizations are unintentional. In practical advice books, like anything else in life, there are no guarantees of results. Readers are cautioned to rely on their own judgment about their individual circumstances and act accordingly.

This book is not intended for use as a source of legal, medical, business, accounting or financial advice. All readers are advised to seek services of competent professionals in the legal, medical, business, accounting, and finance fields.

TABLE OF CONTENTS

INTRODUCTION

Recently, social media posts about natural ways of healing the body are shared a lot more. With the onset of more complicated diseases, many have decided to go back to nature as a way of healing their bodies. The use of essential oils is one popular choice made by a lot of people nowadays. Because of the sudden interest and increasing demand for these oils, many stores are starting to stock up on them. But really, what are essential oils, and why the sudden interest in them?

Actually, the use of essential oils is not new. These oils, otherwise known as aromatic oils in the ancient times, have been in use around the world for centuries. Their use cannot be pinpointed to a single culture, as records show that they have been widely used by different ancient peoples. They used the oils for various purposes, from healing the sick to the fulfillment of certain rituals. It is quite difficult to pinpoint for sure where and when essential oils became popular for healing purposes, but the knowledge of their use became rampant around the world.

The earliest known proof that humans already knew about plants' healing properties was first found in a region of France. Cave paintings suggested that the people used medicinal plants every day. They were carbon dated to as early as 18,000 B.C.E.

OILS AROUND THE WORLD AND IN ANCIENT HISTORY

According to recorded history and evidence, Egyptians already made use of aromatic oils way back since 4500 B.C.E. They are well-known for their use of ointments, cosmetics, and aromatic oils. They made herbal preparations out of different ingredients, and they were used for medicine, perfume, or incense. They were also known to make use of resins, balsams, scented barks, perfumed oils, and spices in a lot of their every day routines. Pastes and oils from plants were made into medicinal cakes, powders, pills, and ointments. During the time when Egyptian priests were powerful, they were the only ones allowed to make use of aromatic oils. Pharaohs also made use of these oils, with their own blends for various purposes, such as war, meditation, love, and a lot more.

It was back in 2697 to 2597 B.C.E. (from recordings) that China first used aromatic oils. The legendary "Yellow Emperor", or Huang Ti, was famous for his book of internal medicine. The book contained uses for some oils, and many practitioners of Eastern medicine today still consider it as a useful guide.

The Ayur Veda is traditional Indian medicine that has a history dating back to three thousand years ago. This practice included the use of essential oils when making healing potions. The writings focused on Vedic medicine lists down more than 700 substances such as ginger, sandalwood, cinnamon, and myrrh as effective ones for healing. When the Bubonic Plague broke out, Ayur Veda was successful in replacing antibiotics that were ineffective. The use of aromatic oils and plants were believed to be not just purely medicinal, but they were also a part of nature that was Godly. It played an important role in the philosophies and spirituality of those who practice Ayurvedic medicine.

The Ancient Greeks also recorded their knowledge of the uses of essential oils that they learned from the Egyptians. This was said to be between

400 to 500 B.C.E. Soldiers took with them ointments made of myrrh to help combat infections. Hypocrites, the Greek physician who is now known as "Father of Medicine", was able to record the effects of about 300 plants such as cumin, thyme, peppermint, saffron, and marjoram. His vast knowledge of plants was of Ayur Vedic origin, and he was able to learn such from the encounters of Greek soldiers traveling with Alexander the Great. Galen was another Greek physician who used plants for medicine.

So, using essential oils is not new. It has been extensively studied even by different cultures before. As Hypocrites once believed, the purpose of a doctor is to naturally wake up the energies of the body that speed up healing. This can be achieved through the use of aromatic oils.

CHAPTER I:
What are Essential Oils and What Can They Do?

Essential oils are natural oils that are found in plants, but are much more concentrated. Essential oils are extracted from plants using a process known as distillation (either by water or steam). Plant bark, leaves, roots, flowers, or stems are used to take out the oils. After the plant parts have been distilled, the result is the essential oil that is very concentrated. It will have the characteristic properties, true essence, and fragrance of the plant it was taken from. This also includes the healing properties of the plant.

While the oils are still in the plant, they serve a variety of purposes. They regularly change their chemical composition in order to help the plant to adapt to changes in the external and internal environment. Here are the different purposes why plants create essential oils:

- To make the plant able to compete with other plants (allelopathy)

  Allelopathy is the natural way that plants ensure that they don't have other plants growing within their area or zone that will compete for nutrients. They do this by releasing chemicals that prevents other plants from growing near them.

- To attract agents of pollination and dispersal

  Insects, much like people, are also attracted to certain types of plants for any of these reasons: color, aroma, or the physical structure (morphology). Insects are the main propagators of pollination for over 200 million years. Studies have shown that the scent of flowers are more ancient attractants to insects than flower color. Butterflies and bees are attracted to the scent of flowers.

- To defend against other animals and insects.

Plants also have their own defense mechanisms to protect themselves from predators. Terpenoid compounds that plants produce deter any animals from going near them. A good example is the peppermint plant. It contains compounds that let insects go away.

- To serve as an antibacterial and antifungal for the plant

Some plants and trees release complex mixtures of terpenes and resins in order to fight against bacteria, fungi, and other microbes. These foreign organisms may threaten the survival of the plants, which is why the plants also have to protect themselves.

Once extracted, essential oils, contrary to their name, do not have an oily texture. They are called as such because they have chemicals that are oil-soluble. Each may contain about 100-200 different chemicals. The combination of various chemicals makes it possible for the essential oils to have their healing and therapeutic properties. This is also why different types of essential oils may also have overlapping effects.

Many essential oils are popular because of their effects on relieving various symptoms and ailments. They have stimulating, detoxifying, anti-depressant, antiviral/antibacterial, calming properties and a lot more. And to make it even better, they are safe, natural, and cost-effective compared to the rising costs of health care. Many people opt to use oils because of the side effects that conventional medications have.

Here are 11 benefits that could be taken from using essential oils:

1) Essential oils can balance one's hormones.

2) They can help fight infections and boost immunity.

3) They support one's digestion.

4) They increase energy levels.

5) They help improve one's brain function.

6) They reduce anxiety and emotion stress.

7) They alleviate pains and aches.

8) They boost hair and skin health.

9) They reduce toxicity in the body, as well as one's home.

10) They help relieve migraines and headaches.

11) They promote better and restful sleep.

Here are 3 examples of well-used and loved essential oils and their benefits:

- Lavender – This oil helps to alleviate panic attacks, anxiety, mental fatigue, and depression. It has also been found to help for stretch marks and bruises.

- Frankincense – This is an immune system stimulator, and it helps alleviate bronchitis, asthma, and coughing.

- Peppermint – This is well-known to help with exhaustion, nausea, and vertigo. This also works well with headaches.

Some people also learned that mixing certain oils together makes their effects even more potent in treating ailments. Read on to find out different ailments that could be solved using essential oils.

CHAPTER 2:
What Ailments Can You Treat Using Essential Oils?

This is dedicated to various ailments and the essential oils that could be used to alleviate them. You can choose any type of essential oil that you may have, or you may also come up with your own blends to maximize the benefits.

1) ACNE

- Tea tree – This oil has antifungal and antimicrobial properties. Tons of over-the-counter treatments for acne have tea tree oil in them, which indicates that it is a popular treatment for acne. To use, add about 2 to 3 drops onto a clean cotton ball and apply on the affected area. This can also be added to body or facial wash, or added to a spray bottle with water and sprayed on affected areas of the face or body.

- Juniper berry – This has natural antimicrobial and antibacterial properties, which is why it is also widely used to treat skin infections and irritations. It also has detoxifying properties that fight off toxins that can cause acne. Put about 2 to 3 drops of oil onto a clean cotton ball and apply onto the affected area/s. For those with sensitive skin, it is best to dilute the oil in some jojoba or coconut oil before applying topically.

- Lavender – The skin will definitely have profound benefits with lavender due its antioxidant and antimicrobial abilities. It can soothe and nourish the skin, which is great for treating acne. It may also reduce the appearance of scars and dark spots due to acne. Lavender oil may be used to de-stress, as stress can cause overproduction of sebum which can lead to acne. You can diffuse about 5 drops of the oil at home, or you can apply topically (back of neck, temples, or wrists). It may also be applied directly on acne-affected areas.

- Clary sage – Clary sage contains an ester called linalyl acetate, which is known to reduce inflammations of the skin. This is a natural remedy for skin irritation, including acne. It also helps regulate the skin's ability to produce oil, as overproduction is associated with skin breakouts. This essential oil also inhibits the growth of bacteria. Apply about 3 drops of clary sage oil and onto the affected areas. This can help fight the bacteria that clogs the pores. For those with sensitive skin, diluting clary sage in jojoba or coconut oil is best. Fill a 5ml bottle with jojoba oil and add 2 drops of clary sage oil. Shake well then apply the mixture onto oily areas, as well as those that are acne-affected.

2) DRY SKIN

- Frankincense – This oil is excellent for dry skin, as it also has anti aging benefits. Adding this to facial toner can help alleviate dry skin. Try adding 2-3 drops of frankincense oil to an unscented lotion or base oil then mix. Apply directly to the skin. Do not apply this to broken skin, but it is okay if the skin is already starting to heal.

- Cedarwood – Cedarwood has astringent properties, which means it helps to absorb excess oil, even dandruff on one's skin. This is best for those who have oily skin, as well as those who have skin infections, spots, or acne. You can add some oil in your soap or skin lotion, and rub on the itchy or affected area directly. You can also put five drops of cedarwood essential oil into your bath and soak in it.

- Sandalwood – This oil is known to be very effective when

treating various skin ailments. It has anti-aging, itch-relieving, skin-softening, and complexion-clearing properties. Mix a few drops of the oil into a base oil and use it to combat areas that have dry skin.

- German chamomile – It has a calming effect, and also does a lot of good for dry skin. It can go deeper into the skin to soothe and hydrate all layers. This is also best for people with sensitive skin. You can blend two drops of this oil in some purified water, put into a spray bottle, and use as a natural skin mist.

- • Geranium – This improves circulation and also reduces inflammation. You can mix 5 drops of geranium oil in a teaspoon of coconut oil and apply onto the affected areas. You can also put 2 drops of oil in your daily body or facial wash.

- Palmarosa – This oil can help to balance the epidermis' ability to create oil. It also fosters regeneration of skin cells, and balances the production of sebum. You can add 2-3 drops of palmarosa oil in bathwater or as massage oil to help with skin problems, like dry skin. You can also blend 2 drops of this oil with coconut oil to serve as a skin moisturizer.

3) AGE SPOTS

- Frankincense – This has anti-inflammatory and anti-infection properties. It also has anti-cancer and anti-tumor properties, making it a good choice for treating age spots, warts, moles, and other skin conditions. You can add a few drops to your moisturizer and use it for places with age spots. You can also put some oil directly on your skin thrice a day to improve the appearance of age and sun spots.

- Helichrysum – This helps in cell regeneration and can help protect against sun radiation. Dilute some of this oil in rosehip seed oil, then massage onto areas with age spots.

- Lavender – This helps foster skin regeneration, making it an excellent oil for treating scars, burns, and age spots. In one ounce of extra virgin olive oil, mix about 10 drops of lavender oil. Use this as a massage oil for your skin every morning, right after you take a shower. Repeat this before sleeping. You can increase the quantities of this as needed.

- Carrot seed – This is also a good essential oil for skin regeneration. Aside from smoothing dry skin, it also helps in lightening age spots and in enhancing the tone of aging skin. Try adding a few drops of this oil to regular massage oil and massage onto your skin. You can also add carrot seed oil to face masks that are anti-aging to boost their capacities.

- Geranium – This helps in regulating sebum production and diminishes the appearance of age spots on the face. It is considered as a natural cytophylactic, which promotes good health for your cells, as well as regeneration. In a teaspoon of olive or coconut oil, mix 5-6 drops of geranium oil. Massage thoroughly onto skin daily, before you go to sleep.

- Sandalwood – This acts as a good skin regenerative and it is a natural skin tonic, making it good for treating age spots. You can directly put some sandalwood essential oil onto areas with your age spots.

- Myrrh – This is essentially great for aging skin, as it can improve skin tone, elasticity, and firmness. It has strong anti-inflammatory properties as well. It has the capacity to protect the skin from the harmful rays of the sun too. As treatment, you can add 2-3 drops of myrrh oil to your body moisturizer or face cream. Apply thoroughly and massage for a minute or two, and do this twice a day.

4) BRUISES

- Lavender – This has been found to reduce the healing time of bruises, especially when it is used together with a compress. It has antiseptic and healing properties. Right after you get injured, put 3 to 5 drops of undiluted lavender essential oil on the area. This will promote healing, prevent bruising, and provide pain relief.

- Helichrysum – Topical application of this oil is said to help lessen visible scars of patients who have undergone cosmetic surgeries. This is also considered as one of the best essential oils to use for hematoma. In order for this oil to be most effective, you only need to apply about 3 to 5 drops directly onto the bruised area. This has to be done about 6 to 12 hours after you get injured.

- Geranium – Known to stimulate the production of new and healthy tissue, it also boosts circulation, especially in the bruised site. It may cause a bit of inflammation at first, but it will hasten healing once it is used regularly. For fast results, mix some geranium oil with a carrier oil such as coconut or jojoba. Apply on the affected area. Avoid using the undiluted form as this could irritate the affected are more.

- Rosemary – This is a usual ingredient for bruise remedies. It has been found that rosemary oil contains bioactive compounds that are responsible for helping bruises to heal faster. Rosemary has anti-inflammatory compounds and antioxidants that help stimulate immune response towards bruises, which in turn reduces inflammation. Blend a few drops of rosemary oil with a carrier oil and apply topically on the bruised site. You can also add some of the essential oil in bath water (warm) then fully submerge the bruised area.

- Frankincense – This oil promotes faster healing of wounds and pain relief. This also promotes relaxation, and is beneficial especially for those who have bruises covering a large area. It contains a component known as boswellia, as well as other compounds to help decrease the inflammation. This oil can be used undiluted, and you can use a few drops to be applied onto the bruise. This is also appropriate to use on children when they also have bruises.

- Lemongrass – Application of lemongrass oil on a bruise will help alleviate the pain. It has analgesic properties. It also has anti-inflammatory properties that help to reduce swelling around the bruised area, which then helps to hasten healing. In a tablespoon of coconut oil, blend about 5 to 6 drops of this oil and massage occasionally onto the affected area. You can do this twice or thrice daily, until the bruising disappears.

5) DANDRUFF

- Rosemary – This has antibacterial and antifungal compounds that help to restore the balance in the scalp. It also increases the circulation in the scalp. Add a few drops of rosemary oil into the shampoo and apply on scalp. Another way is to add some rosemary oil to some virgin coconut oil and use it as a scalp rub. Leave the mixture on the scalp overnight and wash out the next morning.

- Tea tree – This oil has antimicrobial, antiseptic, and antibacterial properties that will help to kill any bacteria, yeast, or other microbes that accumulate on the scalp and build dandruff. When the scalp is itchy and inflamed due to dandruff, tea tree oil can cool and soothe the irritated skin. People with more sensitive skin may have to dilute the oil in a carrier oil like olive, coconut, or jojoba before applying onto the scalp. To use, mix about 6 drops of tea tree oil in ¼ cup of olive oil and massage onto the scalp. Leave it on overnight then wash thoroughly the next morning with warm water.

- Lavender – This oil has antifungal and anti-inflammatory properties that can control the fungus that cause dandruff. It also helps to ease the redness and itchiness of your scalp. It encourages a healthy and germ-free scalp. Mix 8 drops of lavender oil to a carrier oil and leave overnight on your scalp. Lavender essential oils will help to soothe the scalp, and at the same time, encourage you to sleep better and deeply.

- Chamomile – This essential oil is one of the best treatments for flaky scalp or dandruff problems. It can soothe dry and itchy scalps, and at the same time, its anti-inflammatory abilities help lessen redness, swelling, and heat. It also helps regulate sebum, as overproduction will also lead to the thriving of fungus (as it likes oily areas). Mix around 8 to 10 drops with a carrier oil and apply it on the scalp. If you wish to make it as a hair rinse, add 5 to 7 drops of essential oil to one cup of distilled water.

- Eucalyptus – This has antibacterial, anti-fungal, and anti-inflammatory abilities which makes it a good choice as treatment for scalp, skin, and hair issues. This can be used alone, or you may also use another essential oil that helps in treating dandruff. This can be applied directly on the scalp in undiluted for, or it can be mixed together with your shampoo.

- Thyme – This oil has strong anti-fungal and antiseptic properties. It also increases the circulation in the scalp, making it a good choice for dandruff treatment. Put some oil onto your hand and massage it onto your scalp.

- Patchouli – Aside from being an anti-fungal and antimicrobial, this also serves as a good moisturizer. These all help keep the bacteria and yeast from multiplying in the scalp. It can be used directly on the scalp without a carrier oil.

- Peppermint – This has a soothing and cooling sensation. These properties stimulate the growth of hair, and it calms any itchiness and eliminates flakes from the scalp. Take 3 tbsp of olive oil and mix about 6 drops of the essential oil and apply to the scalp. Rub nicely and allow to sit for 2 hours. Rinse off with warm water once done.

6) PSORIASIS

- Tea tree – This has anti-fungal, antibacterial, and antiviral properties. These help boost the immune function of the body. Psoriasis may cause itchiness, and tea tree oil can help to soothe scratched areas. This can ease the inflammation and keep infection at bay. You can use this directly onto the affected areas. If the skin is sensitive, it may be best to mix it with a carrier oil first.

- Bergamot – This has strong antiseptic properties which can help stave off infection, as well as defend the skin from further inflammation and itchiness. One of the biggest dangers of having psoriasis is an increased chance of developing infections due to the cracking and bleeding of rashes (especially when are scratched). Mix an equal amount of a carrier oil (like jojoba oil) and bergamot oil. Gently apply about 3 to 4 drops of the mix to areas that are affected. This can greatly help a person have an itch-free sleep, and better/relieved symptoms the next morning.

- Lavender – This oil can help reduce inflammations and pain due to scratching. It can also soothe the skin. Lavender is also good for reducing anxiety and stress, which are known to possibly trigger the onset of psoriasis. To apply topically to affected areas, you may dilute some of the essential oil in another carrier oil. You can also put a bit of oil into your bathwater to soak your skin. You can also opt to mix some oil with the lotion or moisturizer that you use, or use it with a diffuser.

- Geranium – This is known to stimulate the growth of new cells as well as help damaged tissue to regenerate, this oil is an essential go-to oil for those with psoriasis. This also has anti-inflammatory abilities to take away itching and discomfort. Geranium essential oil can be mixed with coconut oil or aloe vera to further increase its potency to soothe inflamed areas of the skin, as well as stimulate the skin to produce a normal amount of tissue, not an overgrowth.

- Chamomile – Flare ups from psoriasis can be averted by moisturizing the skin right away. By doing so, you are actually soothing the skin, and this helps lessen itchiness. Chamomile has an anti-inflammatory ability, and can take away pain temporarily when it is applied. Chamomile and peppermint oil are usually blended to make a powerful soothing oil for psoriasis. These oils can also be ingested. For topical application, you simply have to put some of the mixture onto the areas that are inflamed, and this can be repeated as often as needed until the redness is gone.

- Clary Sage – Often overlooked by many, this oil has great anti-inflammatory and antiseptic capacities that can keep flare-ups from worsening. It also helps to protect the tiny sores on top of a psoriasis patch from getting infected. You can put 10 drops of the oil into your warm bath water and soak the affected areas. Another option is to soak a washcloth in the oil-infused water, and hold it against painful patches for about 10 to 20 minutes to give time for the oil to work.

- Angelica – This is a very good and powerful detoxifier for the body and skin. It can keep the skin moisturized, soothe any discomforts, and take out any pathogens or environmental toxins that can worsen the symptoms of psoriasis. Blend 1 tablespoon of olive oil and 5 drops of angelica oil together and mix well. Massage the mixture onto your rashes and wait until everything is absorbed.

- Myrrh – This oil has compounds that are helpful in treating psoriasis. It can help to heal any cracks on the skin, as it is a mild astringent. It can also help reduce pain, redness, and take out any possible microbes that can infect the patchy areas. The antioxidants in the oil can also help to reduce flare-ups, as well as regulate the immune response. When having flare-ups that are bad, especially when the skin bleeds or cracks, topically apply around 4 to 5 drops of the oil onto the skin. This can be either undiluted or together with a carrier oil like jojoba oil.

7) HAIR LOSS

- Rosemary – This is deemed as one of the best essential oils to be used for the hair. It increases circulation to the scalp, and gives life to undernourished hair. It also stimulates the follicles found at the scalp, which then help promote hair growth and prevent hair loss. Mix a few drops of rosemary oil with some coconut or olive oil, and apply it onto the scalp. Make sure to leave the mixture for at least 10 minutes, and wash with shampoo. Follow this twice a week in order to reap the best results.

- Cedarwood – This oil is also known to boost hair growth and lessen hair loss. It does these by balancing the glands that produce oil in the scalp. This oil also has antibacterial and anti-fungal abilities, which can treat conditions that contribute to hair loss. To use, mix 2 tablespoons of a carrier oil with some drops of cedarwood oil. Massage onto the scalp and leave for at least 10 minutes before you wash it out.

- Lavender – Lavender contains compounds that help keep the hair healthy and strong. It also has the ability to reduce hyperactivity which makes it a good anti-stress oil, as stress also contributes to hair loss. Mix 3 tablespoons of carrier oil with a few drops of lavender oil and apply it onto the scalp. Leave it for about 10 minutes and then wash it off normally with shampoo. This can be repeated several times a week.

- Peppermint – When applied, this oil leaves a cold, tingling sensation on the skin. This then increases the circulation to the area, which also promotes hair growth. A study discovered that when this oil was used on mice, overall hair growth was improved. To use, mix 2 drops of the oil with a carrier oil. Massage the mixture onto the scalp and leave for 5 minutes. Wash the mixture out with shampoo, followed by your conditioner.

- Tea tree – This oil has antimicrobial and cleansing properties, which help to unplug hair follicles. This can then boost hair growth. Mix 10 drops of the oil with your conditioner or shampoo and use it every day. You can also mix 2 tablespoons of a carrier oil (olive, coconut, or jojoba) with 3 drops of tea tree oil. Apply it onto the scalp and leave for 15 minutes, and then rinse out.

- Ylang-ylang – This is best for those who have non-oily hair and skin. This is best for those who suffer from dry scalps because it can promote sebum production. When the scalp is dry, the hair also becomes brittle and dry. Furthermore, ylang-ylang can improve the texture of the hair and lessen breakage. To use, mix 2 tablespoons of warm carrier oil and 5 drops of ylang-ylang essential oil. Massage the combination onto your scalp and wrap with a warm towel. Leave this on for 30 minutes and then rinse.

8) WEAK, LIFELESS HAIR

All essential oils listed may be used to massage onto the hair (diluted in a carrier oil). It may be left on the hair for an hour or even overnight. It has to be rinsed out the next morning. They may also be added to shampoo or conditioner.

- Lavender – This is effective in lessening hair breakage.

- Peppermint - It stimulates the circulation of blood to the roots of the hair; this is important because the hair is properly nourished. You can add a few drops to your natural conditioner or shampoo.

- Ylang-ylang – In Asia, this is widely used as a scalp stimulant. It helps to treat weak and dull hair by balancing the production of oils in the scalp.

9) BRITTLE OR DULL NAILS

- Lemon – This oil is best for dull nails as it will help nourish the cuticle, and at the same time, strengthen the nail. Yellowish nails will become whiter, too, as this oil has whitening properties. The vitamin C in the oil helps protect the cuticles from infections. As a nail hardener, you can mix 2 drops of lemon essential oil with 2 drops of frankincense, 4 drops of wheat germ oil, 1 drop of wintergreen, and 2 drops of myrrh essential oil. Apply a drop of the mixture daily on your nails. For best results, you can apply it multiple times daily. This can also be made into a moisturizing nail soak. Add 5 drops of lemon oil and 3 tablespoons of olive oil in a small bowl. Wash your nails and hands well then soak your nails into the mixture. Keep the nails soaked for at least 5 minutes.

- Myrrh – This is one of the most common essential oils for nail care as it is very moisturizing for the nails. Regular use will help to prevent brittleness and dryness. To moisturize your nail, fill ¾ of a small roll on bottle with grapeseed oil and add in 5 drops of myrrh essential oil. Mix well then apply on the cuticles daily before you sleep. As a nail strengthener, mix 2 tablespoons of apricot oil with 2 drops of myrrh essential oil. Add in 2 drops each of wheat germ oil and frankincense. Massage the mixture onto your nails two times a week.

- Lavender – One of the safest oils that can be used directly on the nails without the help of carrier oils. It helps to protect nails while at the same time moisturizing and strengthening them. The benefits may be enhanced by mixing 15 drops of the oil with 1 cup of water and 1 tablespoon of olive oil. Soak washed nails in the mixture as long as you need.

11) BAD BREATH

These oils may be made into a natural alcohol-free mouthwash to help get rid of bad breath.

- Peppermint – This oil is at the top of the list for halitosis. The strong aroma and flavor neutralizes the mouth odors. It also has antiseptic properties that prevent plaque and tooth decays as it wards off germs. You can make a mouthwash by mixing 8 drops of peppermint oil to ½ cup hydrogen peroxide. Mix both well then add ½ cup distilled water then stir again. This can be used for a week.

- Spearmint – This oil also comes from the same family as peppermint, and is also a common ingredient in mouth washes and toothpastes. It helps to freshen the breath, and it also maintains good oral health.

- Lemon – This has properties that help deodorize and neutralize bad smells emanating from the mouth. It also boost saliva production, as a dry mouth may also cause bad breath.

12) TOOTH DECAY/GUM DISEASE

- Clove – This oil has anti-inflammatory and antimicrobial properties that make it a great addition to prevent the onset of tooth decay and/or gum disease. It has also been found to decrease plaque with regular use. For an antiseptic mouth wash, mix 1 cup of water and 20 drops of clove essential oil. Shake very well, take a small amount, and swish around for 15-30 seconds then spit. Do this daily.

- Eucalyptus – It has antibacterial and pain-relieving abilities that will help alleviate the pain from toothaches or gum pain. Add into a diffuser about 3-5 drops of essential oil and inhale daily for 30 minutes.

- Cinnamon – This is a great antiseptic because it has great antimicrobial properties. It also prevents dental plaque, especially when used together with clove.

- Oil of Oregano – This is one of the best antibacterial oils for gingivitis. Teeth and gums will be better as it helps alleviate inflammation due to bacteria.

- Tea Tree – This is an effective remedy against sore gums. It has antiseptic properties that help take out bacteria that cause the infection. You can add this oil to your mouthwash.

13) LOSS OF APPETITE

- Peppermint or Ginger – If the loss of appetite is because of nausea, a sniff of these oils can help to lessen the nausea. When the nausea is gone, the person will also feel a lot better and may start eating.

- Lime, Lemon, or Orange – These citrus oils have an energizing effect, which can wake the appetite. Put these in a diffuser and inhale 30 minutes before eating.

- Spearmint – Similar to peppermint, spearmint essential oil is invigorating. They can mentally and physically energize a person, which may also stimulate the appetite. This oil has the ability to work at the cellular level when inhaled.

- Oregano – This is an essential oil that can improve the immune system, reduce nasal congestion and asthma. This has also been found to relax the tension felt in the stomach, which can then increase one's appetite. The oil can be diluted with water and applied on the skin. This can also be taken as hot steam.

14) DIARRHEA

- Peppermint – This is a good oil to relieve stomach cramps due to diarrhea. This oil can invigorate and cool the abdominal area, too. Diluted amounts of food-grade peppermint oil can be ingested to stop diarrhea, too.

- Lemon – This oil has a detoxifying effect that can eliminate viruses, toxins, or bacteria that irritate the stomach. The clean and fresh smell of this oil can also help alleviate nausea when it is inhaled.

- Ginger – This oil has an anti-inflammatory ability, which is a good combatant for diarrhea. It also offers pain relief from stomach cramps that accompany diarrhea. The warm and spicy smell of ginger may help decrease the feelings of lightheadedness and queasiness that are associated with diarrhea.

- Chamomile – This oil has calming properties which can work for diarrhea, too. It is usually used for various blends to reduce inflammation, calm the stomach, and alleviate any stomach cramps.

- Lavender – This is quite similar to chamomile, as it is also calming, and popularly used to treat skin problems. When this oil is diffused, it gives a person a sense of tranquility and peace, which can greatly lessen diarrhea that is anxiety related. Massage this oil on the abdomen to relieve stomach cramps and reduce inflammation.

- Frankincense – This is a healing oil that can fight infections, and it also makes the immune system stronger. By boosting the immune system, diarrhea is resolved a lot faster, too.

- Tea tree – This one of the good essential oils to use if the diarrhea is caused by viruses or bacteria, as it has antibacterial and antiviral properties.

- Oil of oregano – This essential oil is powerful against a lot of microbes: yeast, bacteria, fungi, viruses, etc. When this is ingested, it can kill parasites. There are oil of oregano capsules available that could be taken once daily after meals.

15) WEIGHT LOSS

- Cinnamon – This oil helps to regulate insulin ang blood sugar levels in the body. This can then help lessen overeating and cravings for sugar. Cinnamon can be used by diffusing 5 drops of the oil in a diffuser. You can also mix 1-2 teaspoons of coconut oil with 5 drops of cinnamon and apply it on your chest, wrists, or abdomen.

- Peppermint – This oil may also be used to lose weight, as it helps to curb your appetite. It affects the area in the brain that triggers the feeling that you are full. There has been a study that showed people who sniffed peppermint essential oil every two hours were able to take fewer calories in a day compared to those who don't.

- Lemon – Lemon water has been known to aid in weight loss, and the essential oil is also helpful. This increases energy levels, and it also improves the digestion of fat. It helps with the lymphatic drainage, which then reduces the amount of body wastes that lead to health issues and hinder the body from losing weight. You can diffuse five drops of lemon your diffuser with some water.

- Lavender – This oil has been said to curb any unhealthy cravings you may have. Stress can make you crave fattening comfort food, and lavender will help you to relax and calm down. You can apply 2-3 drops of the oil on your wrists, temples, and back of the neck before you sleep.

- Holy basil – Some researches say that this essential oil can help with regulating anxiety and stress. When the body is stressed, it produces more cortisol, which can trigger weight gain. Add a drop or two into a cup of water (warm) and then drink it.

- Ginger – This oil is known to aid digestion, ease sugar cravings, as well as reduce the inflammation in the body. This is why many restaurants also offer ginger candies, and it is also a good treatment for nausea. Ginger essential oil has thermogenic properties that help boost the metabolism and burn fat. You can try adding 2 drops of the oil in a warm cup of water and drink it like tea. You can also inhale it or add 2-3 drops of the oil into your warm bath water.

- Grapefruit – The Grapefruit became a big thing before, and there may be some backing evidence. Grapefruit essential oil has fat-burning properties. It supports fat breakdown as it activates the different enzymes in the body. It also contains compounds that support the metabolism and clean out the lymphatic glands, making the system more effective in delivering nutrients all throughout the body. Massage some grapefruit oil onto your stomach to reduce the belly fat. You can also put 1-2 drops of the oil in water and drink it to reduce cravings, or apply two drops to your chest or wrists.

16) ACID REFLUX/ GERD (GASTROESOPHAGEAL REFLUX DISEASE)

- Ginger – This essential oil provides a lot of benefits, including cleaning up the body of bad bacteria, boosting the immune system, and preventing the onset of ulcers due to acid reflux. You can take 2 to 4 drops of the oil mixed in 8 ounces of warm water. You can also massage 2 drops of oil on the throat or chest to relax and soothe the muscles.

- Peppermint – This has soothing and relaxing properties that help with acid reflux. However, this must also be used carefully as it can also worsen the condition. A good mix to use for prevention of heartburn or acid reflux is by mixing 2 drops of this oil with 4 drops each of eucalyptus and fennel oils in 2 teaspoons of almond or hazelnut carrier oil. The mixture may then be rubbed onto the throat, chest, and throat.

- Lemon – Though it comes from a sour fruit, lemon essential oil is actually alkaline in nature, and it aids in neutralizing the stomach acid. It is also a mild antibacterial that can take out the bad bacteria in the digestive system. Adding a drop of lemon essential oil to a glass of warm water can help to flush the toxins and leftover acids in the stomach. Do this 30 minutes before a meal, and sip slowly. You may also put 1 to 2 drops on your tongue and swish it with your saliva before swallowing.

- Lavender – This is a staple in aromatherapy, and it works well for heartburn due to its relaxing properties. For those who have night-time acid reflux and insomnia because of GERD, lavender oil will be very helpful. You can massage 1-2 drops of the oil on your chest and belly for relief. You may opt to dilute it first with almond or coconut oil. Therapeutic-grade lavender oil that can be ingested may also be put at the back of the tongue to improve digestion and soothe the stomach. You can also put a drop of oil into some tea and drink after you eat dinner.

17) ABDOMINAL PAIN

- Fennel – This is an effective natural remedy especially for those who have abdominal pain due to gas accummulation in the tummy. Anethole, a component in fennel has an antispasmodic and carminative effect that helps to calm down the intestines' smooth muscles. It can decrease any pain felt at the abdomen. You can put 2 drops in a handkerchief and inhale it, or mix it in some vegetable oil (such as olive oil) and rub your stomach area with it.

- Peppermint – When you suffer from bloating, you can use peppermint essential oil as it relaxes the intestinal muscles. The digestive gases that are stuck inside and cause pain can then pass more quickly. There are readily available peppermint oil capsules that you can take to alleviate the pain.

- Oregano – This oil has anti-inflammatory and antispasmodic abilities. It has long been used in ancient Greece, China, and Egypt to aid with digestion. This can relieve bloating and gas as it soothes intestinal movement. Mix a few drops with a carrier oil and rub it onto the soles of your feet for quicker absorption.

18) MIGRAINES/ HEADACHES

- Peppermint – This is one of the most commonly used essential oils for migraines and headaches. It has menthol which eases pain and helps the muscles to relax. You can dilute the oil with some carrier oil before applying it onto your temples to relieve the pain.

- Rosemary – This oil has powerful analgesic and anti-inflammatory properties. It has been used even a long time to reduce pain, improve circulation, and decrease stress. All of these, when solved, can help headaches. Mix a few drops of the oil with coconut oil or any other carrier oil and massage your head with it.

- Lavender – This is another oil that is commonly used for relaxation, and it has been found to be helpful in treating migraines and headaches. Inhaling the scent can help with the acute management of migraines. Apply diluted lavender essential oil onto the affected area, or use an oil diffuser to inhale the scent. You can also add some oil into your warm water bath.

- Chamomile – This soothes the muscles and relaxes the body, making it one of the best oils for tension headaches. This can also help in treating insomnia and anxiety, both of which may also trigger headaches. You can add a few drops of diluted chamomile essential oil into a bath, or in some hot water so you can inhale the steam.

- Eucalyptus – When you suffer from headaches due to sinus problems, eucalyptus can open up the nasal passages and clear out the sinuses. This can then relieve the sinus tension that is causing the headaches. Mix a drop of this oil with a carrier oil and apply it to your chest. You can also add some drops to some hot water and inhale the steam.

- Camphor – This is a main ingredient found in Vicks, and it has pain-relieving abilities. It also acts as a decongestant, which is helpful for sinus headaches. Mix 1 teaspoon of carrier oil (hazelnut, grapeseed, or olive) with 5 drops of camphor essential oil and apply it to the temples and forehead. For headaches due to congestion, boil 2 to 3 cups of water and add 4 to 5 drops of the oil and inhale the steam.

19) LACK OF ENERGY

- Orange – Citrus oils are known to boost energy and motivation. The energetic scent of orange makes you more focused and productive. This also helps to kick away depression and stress. To use, you can blend some drops of this oil with a couple of drops of water.

- Lemon – Similar to orange essential oil, lemon also helps to perk you up. The fresh scent also serves as a good pick-me-upper during the day.

- Eucalyptus – This oil helps to stimulate the brain and serves to energize you. Keep in mind that you should dilute this essential oil in some carrier oil before use, and never take it orally.

- Grapefruit – This is one of the best energy boosters among the essential oils. It encourages the release of fatty acids in the bloodstream, which makes it possible for the body to turn them into energy.

- Basil – This oil, especially the French basil type, is known to stimulate the adrenal glands, and it helps relieve a person from mental fatigue.

- Neroli – This oil promotes self-confidence, calmness, positivity, and relaxation. Add a few drops to your diffuser and inhale the scent of this oil.

20) INSOMNIA

For the following oils, you can rub an oil of your choice (diluted in a carrier oil) at the bottoms of the feet or back of the neck before sleeping. You can also add a few drops of oil into some water in your diffuser. Be sure to situate it next to your bedside.

- Lavender – This tops the list of essential oils for insomnia. This has been extensively studied, as it improves sleep quality among those who suffer from insomnia.

- Vetiver – When insomnia is due to restless activity of the brain, this oil can help it to calm down, and finally get ready for bed.

If the scent is too strong, you can mix it with another oil such as chamomile or lavender.

- Roman chamomile – This is known to have soothing, calming, and relaxing properties that help to make a peaceful atmosphere inside your bedroom.

- Ylang Ylang – This essential oil can help improve the quality of sleep.

- Bergamot – This can help with emotional balancing, especially when you are suffering from overwhelming emotions. It has a calming ability.

- Marjoram – This is a wonderful oil for joints and muscles, and it helps in making your sleep peacefully.

- Spikenard – This oil may act as a sedative, which is helpful for those with insomnia. Feelings of anxiety and restlessness go away.

21) ANXIETY

The essential oils here may be diluted in some carrier oil first, and then sniffed.

- Lavender – Known as an essential oil that has relaxing and calming effects, it is a restorative for the nervous system. It helps with general nervous tension, irritability, panic attacks, restlessness, and a lot of other anxiety issues.

- Rose – This is the second most popular essential oil for lavender when it comes to treating depression and anxiety. The scent settles down an anxious person. It helps with panic attacks, shock, and grieving.

- Vetiver – The energy given off by vetiver is grounding and tranquil, which is why they use this often for stabilization, self-awareness, and calmness. Vetiver essential oil is a tonic for the nervous system that helps reduce hypersensitivity, shock, and panic attacks.

- Ylang Ylang – This oil has uplifting and calming effects, which makes it a good choice for anxiety. It helps with boosting feelings of happiness and optimism, and it soothes feelings of fear.

22) INFLAMMATION

- German chamomile has pain-relieving and anti-inflammatory compounds. It has also been found to aid joint health.

- Sweet marjoram – The sedative compounds found in this essential oil can help relieve muscle spasms and pain.

- Eucalyptus – This oil has a strong smell, and it contains compounds that have analgesic and anti-inflammatory abilities. It can help with muscle pain and nerve pain.

- Clary Sage – This oil has anti-inflammatory and anti-spasmodic compounds and can soothe the mind and the body. Make sure to use this oil in small amounts as it could be overwhelming in its effectiveness.

- Frankincense – This has a mild sedative effect, but it comes with strong anti-inflammatory compounds. It can relieve general pain and stress.

- Blue Tansy – It has natural pain-relieving and anti-inflammatory compounds, which is why many people have been using this essential oil for years. It has been found to help lower blood pressure, too.

23) COUGH & COLDS

- Eucalyptus – This essential oil works as an expectorant, as it helps to flush out microorganisms and toxins that contribute to sickness. It also helps to dilate the blood vessels and makes it possible for your body to deliver more oxygen into your lungs. This is helpful if you have a cough and/or cold and have trouble catching a breath. You can diffuse 5 drops and inhale the scent before sleeping. It can also be applied topically on the neck and chest to lessen the severity of cough.

- Peppermint – It contains menthol which has antiviral and antibacterial properties, as well as anti-spasmodic and antitussive ones. It helps to improve the nasal flow of air especially when your sinuses are congested, as it helps to unclog them. Peppermint also helps to take away throat itchiness. Diffuse about 5 drops at work or home, then inhale it directly. You can also apply 2-3 drops on your chest, temples, and back of the neck.

- Rosemary – It relaxes the smooth muscle of the trachea, which relieves cough. It can reduce coughing fits, and it also works to boost your immune system naturally. Diffuse 5 drops or mix half a teaspoon of coconut oil with 2 drops of the oil and rub onto your chest.

- Lemon – This supports lymphatic drainage and boosts the immune system, both of which can help you to recover from coughs and colds faster. It has antioxidant, anti-inflammatory, and antibacterial properties, too. Diffuse 5 drops, and you can even add some eucalyptus oil to make it even better.

- Oregano – Carvacrol and thymol, two ingredients in oregano oil, have antifungal and antibacterial properties. Due to these properties, oregano has been found to be a natural alternative to the use of antibiotics for respiratory problems. You can combine 2 to 3 drops of oregano essential oil with the same amount of a carrier oil and apply topically on your back, chest, neck, or at the soles of your heart. You can also diffuse 3 to 5 drops at work or home.

24) DEPRESSED IMMUNE SYSTEM

- Lemon – This has great detoxifying effects and can help to boost the immune system. You can add a bit of lemon essential oil in your water to cleanse and clear out the toxins in your body.

- Thieves – This is a natural immune booster as it has antibacterial and antifungal properties. You can mix a drop of thieves oil with some carrier oil and apply it to areas of your body that need a boost. You can also inhale the scent by putting a few drops into a diffuser.

- Peppermint – This oil can help your body detoxify, which can then boost your immune system response.

- Lavender – This supports better sleep, which then helps your body to restore and heal. When your body is well-rested, your immune system will work a lot better, too. You can rub some on the soles of your feet or diffuse the oil.

- Valor – This also helps you to sleep better, and it also boosts confidence. When you are feeling under the weather, you can use this oil so that you can rest better. Diffuse some drops to reap the benefits.

25) WARTS

- Oregano – One of the most effective and fastest treatments for warts, it is considered a "hot" oil. It can irritate the skin and cause a burning sensation, which is the best to burn off any warts, including very stubborn ones.

- Lemongrass – This has been studied before, and results showed that it can get rid of the herpes simplex 1 virus, which is the cause of cold sores. It is also a good treatment for shingles, which is caused by the same virus that triggers chicken pox.

- Tea tree – This is also a good essential oil for warts as it has antiviral compounds. It doesn't work as fast as oregano or lemongrass oils, but it is still very effective in treating warts.

- Manuka – This has antiviral properties that also help to stop the spread of some viruses, given that it is applied as early as possible. For maximum benefits, apply this essential oil as soon as you notice the appearance of a wart.

- Cajeput – This is an essential oil that is taken from the same family as that of tea tree, and it has antiviral properties. When combined with tea tree, this is an effective treatment for warts.

26) DECREASED LIBIDO

These oils may be used as topical applications, diffusions, or sprays.

- Rose – This is a calming and anxiety-relieving oil, and it also acts as an aphrodisiac. The scent is usually associated with romance, and it helps to entice people, and in turn, increases libido.

- Jasmine – This oil has been found to increase alertness and arousal, especially when applied topically. This may be used as a sensual massage oil or perfume.

- Clary Sage – When the libido dips because of hormonal shifts such as in menopause, clary sage can balance that. It also has an anti-depressant effect on women in menopause. You inhale or diffuse in order to balance the hormones, relax, or get yourself in the mood.

- Ylang Ylang – This oil is a well-known aphrodisiac in the world of aromatherapy. The gentle smell is appealing to almost everyone. It can be used as a massage oil, or used for diffusion or inhalation.

- Neroli – A clinical trial found out neroli oil inhalation can increase sexual desires, relieve symptoms of menopause, and reduce blood pressure. This is extremely helpful for those who have low libido.

- Fennel – This oil has been found to increase the libido, alleviate symptoms of dysmenorrhea, promote menstruation, increase milk production, and even facilitate birth. This has estrogenic effects, which is a good addition to blends that increase the libido. You can use fennel oil together with massage oils or lotion.

27) DEPRESSION

- Bergamot – This is a very stimulating type of oil, which is why it makes a great anti-depressant. It creates feelings of energy, joy, and freshness, and it does that by boosting circulation. It has the ability to work as an anti-anxiety treatment, too. Rub 2-3 drops of the oil on your hands and cup them over your nose and mouth. Breathe in slowly.

- Lavender – This has long been used to treat depression as it serves to lift up the mood. Compared to conventional medications for depression, lavender oil does not have adverse side effects. A study also found that lavender is also great for those who are suffering from PTSD (post traumatic stress disorder). The oil may be diffused next to your bed. A few drops of the oil may be rubbed behind the ears.

- Roman Chamomile – This is a good essential oil that promotes relaxation and fights stress. It soothes your emotions, which is a good thing for depression.

- Ylang Ylang – This oil helps to prevent depression and the onset of negative emotions that are related or associated with the said condition. Inhaling this oil can have immediate effects for the mood.

28) ULCERS

- Carrot Seed – This has antibacterial, anti-fungal, and antioxidant properties. It reduces the effects of pylori cateria inside the stomach. This bacteria is known to cause stomach upsets, including ulcers.

- Cinnamon Bark – This essential oil has "eugenol", a compound that is found to heal stomach ulcers. This compound also helps to lessen pain from stomach ulcers. The oil also helps to restore the balance of the natural flora in the instestines and it also fights against pathogens.

- Lemongrass – This oil has been proven to be effective in fighting against bacteria that are drug-resistant. It also has the ability to slow down the growth of pylori bacteria. This is why it is effective in treating gastric ulcers. It helps to reduce pain and inflammation.

- Clove – This is a known essential oil that can address different stomach disorders, including ulcers. It has great antibacterial properties, as well as anti-inflammatory abilities. You can apply this topically to help soothe stomach ulcers and for pain relief.

- Manuka – This is a cousin of tea tree, and it is a stronger anti-microbial agent, especially against different drug-resistant bacteria. It is an anti-inflammatory as well, as it brings pain relief from peptic ulcers. It also is an anti-spasmodic.

29) SUNBURN

- Lavender – This oil has antibacterial, carminative, and antifungal properties that make it very useful in treating sunburn and other skin problems. Mix 1 drop of this oil with aloe vera gel and apply on the affected areas. This will serve as immediate relief. If the area is large, mix some oatmeal in a tub of warm water and 7 to 8 drops of the oil. You can then soak yourself in this.

- Sandalwood – This oil has cooling properties and may be used to calm down inflammation due to sunburn, soothe burns, and even get rid of tans that are uneven. It may also help get rid of microbes that can trigger infection. To use sandalwood for sunburn, you can mix 1 drop of turmeric essential oil (as it has antiseptic properties), 1 to 2 drops of sandalwood, and 30 grams of coconut oil. Apply on affected areas.

- Frankincense – This oil helps to nourish the skin that has been damaged. It rejuvenates the skin and provides hydration, as sunburnt skin will most likely be painful and dry. Mix 1 to 2 drops of frankincense oil with aloe vera gel and apply on the affected areas.

- Peppermint – It is a cooling agent, and the menthol in the oil helps to numb the pain of sunburn. Mix 1 to 2 drops of the oil with 1 to 2 teaspoons of aloe vera gel. Apply on affected areas to soothe the burns.

- Eucalyptus – This oil has pain-relieving and anti-inflammatory properties that can help heal sunburn faster. It also has antibacterial properties that protect the sunburnt parts from getting infected. Mix a cup of water, 1 teaspoon of aloe vera gel, and 2 to 3 drops of eucalyptus oil and transfer to a clean spray bottle. Before going to bed, shake the mixture and spray it onto affected areas. You may also mix some water with 4-5 drops of oil and soak a towel in it. Dab the affected areas with the towel.

30) BUG BITES

- Lemongrass – This has anti-inflammatory and anti-microbial properties. It may help to stop infection when applied.

- Peppermint – This oil helps to reduce itching by a big margin, and this is extremely helpful in lessening the urge to scratch and speeds up the time to heal. It's smell may also deter bugs and can cool and soothe the affected area.

- Basil – This oil has a natural anti-microbial property, and it can stop the growth of bacteria on the bug bite site. It also acts as an insecticide, which reduces the risk of getting more bug bites.

- Tea Tree – This essential oil has anti-itch, antibacterial, and anti-inflammatory properties that all contribute to faster wound healing. It helps to reduce the spread of bacteria, and minimizes swelling.

- Lavender – This serves as an analgesic and it calms down a person who has been bitten.